Healthy Exercises for Seniors and Non-Athletes

Martin Eisen, Ph.D.

Preface

For over sixty years, I have taught and studied Shotokan Karate, Aikido, Kwong Sai Jook Lum Mantis Kung Fu, Yang Tai Chi; Qigong and helped teach Yoga. During this time these arts have become mere shells of their original system, simplified and mixed, like chop suey. One reason is that in modern times few people have the time, interest or perseverance to study a classical art. Another is that to make a profit, you cannot criticize students, make them perform many boring repetitions, but must amuse them,

Even prestigious medical centers, hospitals and universities offer these simplified activities for health, like Yoga, Tai Chi and Qigong (pronounced Chi Kung). They seem to have little knowledge of these original arts or know how to find genuine masters for teachers.

Many teachers are well-meaning and follow their teacher's methodology, not realizing that their teachers really have little knowledge of their art. One purpose of this book is to describe classical Yoga, Tai Chi and Qigong to encourage interested teachers to further their knowledge in order to preserve these systems and prevent further degradation.

Medical professionals should read this book in to learn about Yoga, Tai Chi and Qigong not only to be able to find competent teachers, but also to know which art to recommend. For example, few Yoga teachers are versed in anatomy and physiology and so a physical therapist rather than a Yoga teacher should be recommended. Also, modern Yoga is not suitable for many seniors. A Medical Qigong Doctor should be recommended for serious illnesses and not the feel good Qigong class conducted at many hospitals.

Finally, seniors and non-athletes will learn that vigorous and long duration exercises are not necessary for health. There are non-strenuous activities that can preserve health and also help cure illness – like Tai Chi and Qigong. Students will learn about these arts to help them find knowledgeable teachers. For example, read the Appendix on basic Tai Chi principles and see if a class is doing these.

Contents

Chapter 1

Can Exercise Be Healthy Dangerous Or Help Lose Weight?

Excellent physical condition is not equivalent to good health. Arnold Schwarzenegger needed to have a heart valve replaced. Jean-Claude Van Damme, a famous martial arts actor, suffers from a hearing loss.

Chronic training for and competing in extreme endurance events such as marathons, ultra marathons, ironman distance triathlons, and very long distance bicycle races, can cause transient acute volume overload of the atria and right ventricle, with transient reductions in right ventricular ejection fraction and elevations of cardiac biomarkers, all of which return to normal within 1 week. Over months to years of repetitive injury, this process, in some individuals, may lead to patchy myocardial fibrosis, particularly in the atria, interventricular septum, and right ventricle, creating a substrate for atrial and ventricular arrhythmias. Additionally, long-term excessive sustained exercise may be associated with coronary artery calcification, diastolic dysfunction, and large-artery wall stiffening (1).

The review by Wilhelm, M., in European Journal of Preventive Cardiology, 02/05/2013, focuses on the prevalence, risk factors, and mechanisms of atrial fibrillation (AF) in endurance athletes, and possible therapeutic options. The sports cardiologist should be aware of the distinctive features of AF in athletes. Therapeutic recommendations should be given in close cooperation with an electro-physiologist. Reduction of training volume is often not desired and drug therapy not well tolerated. An early ablation strategy may be appropriate for some athletes with an impaired physical performance, especially when continuation of competitive activity is intended.

Running is more stressful on the body than walking and so is not recommended for the non-athlete. Especially, since walking produces similar health benefits to running. A study (2) used the National Runners' (n=33 060) and Walkers' (n=15 945) Health Study cohorts to examine the effect of differences in exercise mode and thereby exercise intensity on coronary heart disease (CHD) risk factors. It was discovered that equivalent energy expenditures by moderate (walking) and vigorous (running) exercise produced similar risk reductions for hypertension, hypercholesterolemia, diabetes mellitus, and possibly CHD.

Any type of exercise that requires a movement to be repeated many times can also lead to repetitive strain injuries and eventually arthritis.

Lifting more than half your body weight can raise your systolic pressure to 370 millimeters mercury. (Normal systolic pressure is below 120 and normal diastolic pressure, measured as the heart rests between beats, is below 80.). The increased pressure may cause an aortic dissection, in which the heart's main artery tears. This requires immediate surgical intervention to stem blood loss resulting in death (3).

The Nov. 14, 2012, online issue of the J. of the Amer. College of Cardiology contains a paper about the effects of moderate exercise. Certain biomarkers, which were tied to heart injury that was otherwise undetectable but was associated with a higher risk of death by cardiovascular disease, were used. The study consisted of 2900 subjects over the age of 65. They were tracked for their biomarkers along with their levels of physical activity.

The researchers concluded that not only did the biomarkers lower as physical activity went up, but even moderate amounts of exercise in seniors, dramatically lowered the risk of death by heart attack.

Data from the Alzheimer's Association (4) show that: more than five million Americans are living with the disease; one in eight older Americans have it and it's the sixth leading cause of death.

A new report, prepared for the Ontario Brain Institute in Canada (5), has shown that one in seven cases of Alzheimer's disease in Ontario could be prevented if people got some exercise - only 30 minutes per day. The researchers reached this conclusion by studying over 900 recent Alzheimer's and dementia articles, focusing on older adults with and without dementia. The 30-minute a day recommendation didn't even have to be done all at once. It could be broken into three 10-minute intervals throughout the day! Simply walking or doing some other light form of exercise was enough.

One of the reasons why so many of the elderly get Alzheimer's is that 60% of the population age 65 and up are inactive.

Daily activity can also improve depression amongst Alzheimer's patients and makes it easier to cope with daily tasks. Research has shown that physical activity engages the brain to create new neurons and blood vessels.

Whether we gain, lose or maintain body weight is dependent upon three things: the number of calories: required to maintain life (our metabolism), burned through activity, and consumed.

According to Macdonald's calorie chart the calories in the following foods are: Big Mac 570, Large French Fries 540, Coca-Cola Classic 410, Salad 35 and Dressing 160. The total calories in such a meal are 1715. Two such similar meals would contain 3,430 calories.

A 150 lb. person sitting for 15 hours (eating, driving, studying, watching television, etc.) burns an average of about 130 calories an hour. Hence 15 hours of sitting would burn 1,950 calories. If you sleep for 8 hours, you would burn about 552 calories. Exercising by vigorous cycling (14-15.9 mph) for an hour would burn about 704 calories. The total calories burned in a day would be 3,104. Few people can or want to engage in such vigorous exercise.

Thus, diet and not exercise is the primary factor in losing weight.

Obese people can lose weight, probably due to the increased rate of metabolism, by practicing Senobi breathing. This breathing technique, which is simple to learn and only requires 1 minute of practice before each meal, will be discussed in a following chapter. Breathing exercise can also help a benign, enlarged prostate and arrhythmias and will be described in Chapter 6.

Healthful activities often recommended for non-athletes, the sedentary and the elderly are: Yoga, Tai Chi and Qigong (pronounced Chi Kung). Qigong is a Chinese mind/body/breath coordination exercise. These will be discussed in the following chapters to help readers decide which of these they might like. The reader will be made aware of the classical purpose of these activities and the difficulty in finding a classical Master. Then, they can decide if they want to learn the made up, shortened versions, devised for profit or the classical ones.

References

1. O'Keefe, J.H. et al. Potential Adverse Cardiovascular Effects from Excessive Endurance Exercise. Mayo Clinic Proceedings, June 2012.
2. Williams, P. T. and Thompson, P. D. Walking Versus Running for Hypertension, Cholesterol, and Diabetes Mellitus Risk Reduction. Arteriosclerosis, Thrombosis, and Vascular Biology, 04/17/2013 Clinical Article.
3. Intense Weight Lifting Linked to Fatal Heart Trouble. http://www.lifeclinic.com/fullpage.aspx?prid=516325&type=1
4. Alzheimer's Association, "Alzheimer's facts and figures," Alzheimer's and Dementia: The Journal of the Alzheimer's Association March 2012; 8: 131â 168.[WP1].
5. Hauch, V., "Physical activity can prevent Alzheimer's, report finds," The Toronto Star March 2013. http://www.thestar.com/life/health_wellness/2013/03/08/physical_activity_can_prevent _alzheimers_report_finds.html

Chapter 2

What is Yoga? Yoga Therapy?

Most people have erroneous ideas about classical Yoga. Yoga was a spiritual discipline. There were moral precepts and prohibitions that disciples had to follow. In addition, there could be dietary restrictions. Yoga had other paths to enlightenment besides asanas (forms or postures), breathing and meditation, such as, prayer, faith and knowledge. The chosen path was determined by the Guru after analyzing the individual. In some instances any form or exercise was contraindicated. No connection to physical conditioning or health appears in the Vedic literature. You could not pay for Yoga lessons and only received new instructions when your Guru thought you had made sufficient progress. See-

http://en.wikipedia.org/wiki/Yoga

Be cautious about recommending so-called Yoga to patients, especially the elderly. Patients with injuries from practicing Yoga are a common occurrence in our Traditional Chinese Medicine clinic (Arch Acupuncture and Health Center, Philadelphia, PA). Many teachers have made-up their own style ranging from almost no stretching to extreme contortions, not holding postures, practicing in a sauna-like room, using weights, etc. You can injure yourself – see

http://www.nytimes.com/2012/01/08/magazine/how-yoga-can-wreck-your-body.html?_r=1&pagewanted=all

Generally, scientists have little knowledge of Yoga and so cannot select qualified teachers for their subjects. The sample size is frequently too small and there is no control group. For example, recent research shows that regular, moderate stretching improves sport's performance, probably by increasing muscle strength. A control group that just stretches could be used. Finally, experiments are difficult to duplicate because many teachers have their own style.

Another reason why such clinical trials are difficult to evaluate is the subjects are not tracked daily. Anyone who has taught any subject that requires daily practice knows that some people do not practice at home while others are fanatical. In addition, the pupil's report of the amount of daily practice is often erroneous.

The rational use of "Yoga" as a therapy requires a diagnosis based on some underlying theory. A reasonable approach is to use the theory of Ayurvedic medicine, just as Qigong relies on Traditional Chinese Medicine theory. This viewpoint is discussed in

http://www.banyanbotanicals.com/yoga/yogaandayurveda/

Postures should be individually assigned after an Ayurvedic diagnosis. This requires training in Ayurvedic medicine to examine the patient. The diagnosis consists of a past medical history, looking, feeling, questioning the patient and examining the patient. This includes Ayurvedic pulse taking. Then you must know the effects of the postures in Ayurvedic terms (pitta, vata, kapha) in order to select proper postures. The same procedure should be used for selecting proper breathing and meditation exercises.

Finally, to satisfy western doctors, the results should be explained in terms of western science.

Chapter 3

Are You Really Studying Tai Chi and is it Effective for Stress and Health?

1. What is Classical Tai Chi?

Only the Yang style will be discussed. However, similar types of training were used in other classical styles (Chen, Wu and Sun), since these were also internal forms of Kung Fu for health and self-defense. These styles have also been altered and shortened.

The original (old) Yang Tai Chi form was devised by Yang Lu-Chan (1799 – 1872) and consisted of about 128 postures, not counting repetitions. It had both fast and slow movements in it. One of the purposes of the fast movements was to teach fa-jing, small, explosive movements to generate tremendous power in punches, kicks, etc., for self-defense. The (new) long form, practiced by most Yang stylists today, was derived from the Yang Lo – Sim form by Yang Cheng – Fu (1883 – 1936). He removed the fast fa-jing moves, all leaping kicks and made slightly different moves the same. It has about 108 postures. To learn the original form properly took about 5 or 6 years.

Each move in the old form not only showed how to strike acupoints, but the proper direction for striking them, with devastating results. This could result in death of an adversary and was known as Dim Mak.

However, learning the form was not enough for combat and so the following two-person exercises are practiced to learn how to attack and counter. Martial Push Hands (Toi Sau), consisting of countering punches, strikes, kicks, locks and throws (Chin Na). This is not the same as the modern, popular push hands, whose purpose is to push the opponent off-balance. Chi Sau (sticky hands) are also practiced, as well as Pushing Feet, in which only the feet are used to attack and defend. These exercises are mainly to train the student to combat single attacks.

More complex exercises are used for continuous attacks, such as Da Lu (the Great Repulse) and Small San Sau (Free Hands). These exercises only use a small number of the techniques from the old form.

Students then learn Pauchui (Cannon Fist), the remaining movements from the old form, done powerfully rapidly. Pauchui consists of two different formulas, a fixed sequence of moves, which are practiced alone. Later, one student does one formula, while his opponent does the other so that they can practice a sequence of attacks and counters (Large San Sau) without stopping between techniques. At first, they practice slowly and then, gradually faster, with full power. Later, the techniques are applied randomly, leading to free sparring. Usually the Large San Sau is not taught until a student has practiced for at least four years.

Weapons, such as the sword, spear, are also taught as solo forms and then, two-person sparring exercises.

There are several associated medical and health aspects in Tai Chi connected with the old solo form associated martial training exercises. There is a natural, biorhythmic Qi flow in the body every 24 hours, known as the Horary Cycle. In the Horary Cycle, the Qi makes its way through the meridians with its associated organ so that there is a two-hour period during which it is at maximum energy. The order of flow and the maximum energy time periods are:

Lung (3-5 AM) → Large Intestines (5-7 AM) → Stomach (7-9 AM) → Spleen (9-11 AM) → Heart (11AM – 1PM) → Small Intestines (1-3 PM) → Bladder (3-5 PM) → Kidney (5-7 PM)→ Pericardium (7-9 PM) → Triple Energizer (9-11 PM) → Gallbladder (11PM – 1AM) → Liver (1 – 3 AM) → Lung …..

Performing the old Yang form causes your Qi to flow through the Horary Cycle 3 times, energizing the body and helping balance your Qi flow. In addition, each posture in the Yang form can be practiced alone as a Qigong exercise to treat various conditions in the body –for example, holding the single whip posture is beneficial to the joints. In addition, greater difficulty than normal in doing a certain posture can be used to diagnose diseases.

Most people cannot learn to relax sufficiently by only doing the solo form. Practicing the two-person exercises is required. In addition, practicing the San Sau form can energize the practitioners if the acupoints are struck lightly.

In classical Tai Chi, the goal was not to just to make students warriors, but also healers. Dim Mak is not studied just for self-defense to injure people. Techniques for resuscitating attackers and treating accidental practice injuries must also be learned. Moreover, the same Dim Mak technique, when done gently and with a healing mind –set can be used to treat diseases.

Auxiliary Qigong training, which includes holding postures, is also an integral part of training. This helps students increase their internal energy, learn to feel Qi, helps relaxation, rooting, and projecting Qi. External Qi healing is also taught.

Classical Tai Chi takes years of dedicated study. It is very difficult to learn in modern times because of many distractions. To teach Tai Chi to the masses, several different shorter versions of the new, long, Yang Ching – Po have been devised such as: the Beijing 24 movement version, Chen Man-Ching 37 movement form, the 42 movement competition form developed by the Chinese National Wushu Association, and a 48 movement Yang style version by the Chinese National Athletic Association. There is even a fast set version developed by Master Dong Ying-jie.

Practicing the old Yang style probably has more health benefits than practicing a modern, shorter version simply because there are more varied movements in the old form. It is unlikely that the short form causes the Qi to flow 3 times through the Horary Cycle, because different movements influence the Qi flow in different ways and many movements are omitted. There are also many principles (See the Appendix) for doing the postures correctly. In some modern, shorter versions, these principles are not obeyed. Even if the student is taught the principles and has them memorized, it takes years before they can be performed correctly.

Tai Chi research is usually not done on all parts classical Tai Chi as described above, but only some shortened version or even a few postures from some solo form. The results should really be entitled the effects of trying to learn Tai Chi, since the research is usually carried out for months and not years. Beginning students are not doing real Tai Chi and so using a control group that danced or walked might give similar results as doing Tai Chi (9). Further studies, using a walking control group as in (21), should be done.

The Chinese medical health benefits, such as the Horary Cycle effect and postures used as Qigong, have been passed on from Master to student without explanation or justification in terms of traditional Chinese medical theory. Clinical trials have not been carried out to justify all of these claims.

2. Is Tai Chi a Form of Qigong?

The movements in the solo Tai Chi form cause the Qi (internal energy) to circulate. A Tai Chi expert can feel the Qi circulate and after years of practice the circulation of Qi produces the movements. Thus, Tai Chi can be considered to be a form of Qigong according to the Qi definition of Qigong (1).

Even some beginners claim to feel Qi or some of its manifestations. However, often this is just the result of muscle tension restricting blood flow and brainwashing by the instructor. Initially, because beginners must concentrate on the postures and principals, their minds are too preoccupied to feel Qi. Electrical sensations in the back, legs and arms, may be an indication of multiple sclerosis (MS) and not an indication of Qi flow in vital energy channels (2). "The common form of Lhermitte's sign, which occurs in about a third of multiple sclerosis (MS) patients, consists of a feeling of an electric current moving down the back to the legs on flexion of the neck. The spread of the sensation is usually downwards, terminating either at the lower end of the spine or passing down both legs. However, all four limbs may be affected or less frequently the arms alone. Even in the absence of any other symptoms or signs, Lhermitte's sign is a strong indication of MS. In our patient electrical sensation compatible with Lhermitte's sign occurred during bow stance (cervical extension) and push hand practicing (flexion). These positions represent the classical postures of flexion or extension that are associated with Lhermitte's sign. They evoke, due to mechanical deformation of the cord impulses in demyelinated, sensory fibers."

The first definition of Qigong is not suitable for research, since the exact nature of Qi is unknown. However, Tai Chi is a self-training technique or process that integrates the body posture, breathing, and mentality into oneness to achieve the optimal state for both body and mind. Thus, Tai Chi is a form of Qigong according to the second definition in (1).

3. Tai Chi for Relieving Stress

Sandlund and Norlander (3) reviewed more than 20 studies published from 1996 to 1999 on the effects of Tai Chi on stress response and well-being and concluded that, although the slow-movement Tai Chi may not achieve aerobic fitness, it could enhance flexibility and overall psychological well-being. Tai Chi exercises led to an improvement of mood. The researchers concluded that all studies on the benefits of Tai Chi have revealed positive results and that Tai Chi was an effective way to reduce stress.

Wang, Collet, and Lau (4) reviewed general health outcomes of Tai Chi. Among the six studies they reviewed with psychological measures, five reported positive or significant effects of Tai Chi on reducing stress and anxiety. However, biases existed in some of the studies, and it was difficult to draw firm conclusions about the benefits reported. Therefore, more well-designed studies are needed in the future.

The review (5) states that the majority of studies on Tai Chi conducted between 1996 and 2004 had focused on health and well-being of Tai Chi exercise for senior adults. The results show that Tai Chi may lead to improved balance, reduced fear of falling, increased strength, increased functional mobility, greater flexibility, and increased psychological well-being, sleep enhancement for sleep disturbed elderly individuals, and increased cardio functioning.

Jin (7) conducted one of the first studies to examine the effects of Tai Chi (new long Yang and Wu forms) on the endocrine system. Changes in psychological and physiological functioning following participation in Tai Chi were assessed for 33 beginners (8 months or less experience) and 33 practitioners (more than a year's experience). The variables in the three-way factorial design were experience (beginners vs. practitioners), time (morning vs. afternoon vs. evening), and phase (before Tai Chi vs. during Tai Chi vs. after Tai Chi). Phase was a repeated measures variable. Relative to measures taken beforehand, practice of Tai Chi raised heart rate, increased noradrenaline excretion in urine, and decreased salivary cortisol concentration. Relative to baseline levels, subjects reported less tension, depression, anger, fatigue, confusion and state-anxiety, they felt more vigorous, and in general they had less total mood disturbance.

Heart rate for practitioners was higher than that for beginners. Jin attributes this effect to the lower stance and more controlled form of experienced practitioners.

The data suggest that Tai Chi results in gains that are comparable to those found with moderate exercise. There is need for research concerned with whether participation in Tai Chi has effects over and above those associated with physical exercise. A later paper by Jin (9) investigated this query.

The study (9) compares the stress-reducing attributes of Tai Chi to those of brisk walking, meditation, and sitting and reading. There was no difference in the magnitude of cortisol reduction between the Tai Chi group and the other three groups. Hence, an additive effect of the physical exercise component and the cognitive exercise component in the practice of Tai Chi is not evident.

4. Tai Chi for Stress-related Symptoms

Control of Hypertension

In Wang et al.'s recent review (4) of Tai Chi, four studies (two with randomized control) were discussed in terms of its effects on hypertension, and all of them reported that it significantly decreased blood pressure among hypertensive patients.

The results in (11) suggest that light activity and moderate intensity aerobic exercise have similar effects on BP in previously sedentary elderly individuals. If future trials with large sample size and a no-exercise control group confirm these results, promoting light intensity activity could have substantial public health benefits as a means to reduce BP.

This study (13) examined the effects of Tai Chi vs. aerobic exercise for victims of heart attacks, comparing them to a cardiac support group as control. Resting heart rate declined in the Tai Chi group, but curiously, not in the aerobics group in this study. Both the Tai Chi and aerobics groups showed a drop on systolic blood pressure, but only the Tai Chi group showed a drop in diastolic blood pressure.

Improvement of Cardiovascular Conditions

Wang et al. (4) reviewed 16 studies of Tai Chi in patients with cardiorespiratory conditions and reported that its regular practice will delay the decline of cardiorespiratory function in older adults and might be prescribed as a suitable exercise.

One of the few studies to focus on serious Tai Chi practitioners, mostly people in their 60's, who had been practicing the new Yang Long form for 3-10 years, appears in (10). They practiced 3-7 times a week, with an average frequency of 5 times a week. A fairly rigorous practice: 20 minutes of warm-up exercises, 24 minutes of practicing the form paced by the Master, and 10 minutes of cool-down. This study compares these Tai Chi practitioners to a group of sedentary peers matched for age and body size, and looks at cardiorespiratory declines over a two-year period. It has some heart rate profiles that seem to indicate moderate aerobic benefit in older practitioners (this benefit has not been demonstrated in younger subjects).

In (12), changes in heart rate and electrocardiogram were recorded by telemetry in 100 volunteers who were regularly doing a Yang simplified (short) form. During the exercise, the change in heart rate was not very marked and no important electrocardiographic changes were recorded. Thus, it was speculated that the possible beneficial effect of Tai chi on the cardiovascular system cannot be attributed solely to the amount of exercise provided by Tai Chi and additional mechanisms must be sought. The author notes that "16 male and 10 female hypertensives reported a gradual normalization in blood pressure cutting the need for medication entirely or reducing the doses."

The study (18) concluded that Tai Chi was a culturally appropriate mind-body exercise for older adults with cardiovascular risk disease factors. Statistically significant psychosocial benefits were observed over 12-weeks. Further research examining Tai Chi exercise using a randomized clinical trial design with an attention-control group may reduce potential confounding effects, while exploring potential mechanisms underlying the relaxation response associated with mind-body exercise. In addition, future studies with people with other chronic illnesses in all ethnic groups are recommended to determine if similar benefits can be achieved. The authors were unaware of an earlier study (19) on the beneficial effects of Tai chi for dialysis patients.

This research (21) compared the effects of a short style of Tai Chi versus a brisk walking training program on aerobic capacity, heart rate variability (HRV), strength, flexibility, balance. They found Tai Chi to be an effective way to improve many fitness measures in elderly women over a 3-month period It was also significantly better than brisk walking in enhancing certain measures of fitness, including lower extremity strength, balance and flexibility, psychological status, and quality of life.

Twenty patients with coronary heart disease were recruited for the study (28). Ten patients practiced supervised Tai Chi training once a week and home-based Tai Chi training three times a week, together with conventional cardiac rehabilitation for one year. The control group only received the conventional cardiac rehabilitation. The patients in the Tai Chi group showed statistically significant improvement in baroreflex sensitivity. The researchers concluded that Tai Chi training is beneficial in the treatment of coronary heart disease.

Reduction of Chronic Pain Syndrome and Arthritis Symptoms

Pain and fatigue significantly decreased in the experimental group in (14). However, the improvement in daily life performance of the rheumatoid arthritis patients was not statistically significant but their sense of balance was enhanced significantly.

Sun-style Tai Chi exercise (6) was found as beneficial for women with osteoarthritis to reduce their perceived arthritic symptoms and to healthier behavior.

In the short term study (15), the beneficial outcomes for Tai Chi group and aquatic group were significantly better than the self-help group. Tai Chi may be more suitable than aquatic exercise for osteoarthritis. Further longitudinal studies are necessary to confirm these results. Similar conclusions were reached in another study (16) comparing Tai Chi and an aquatic group for rheumatoid arthritis.

The results (17) suggest Tai Chi does not exacerbate symptoms of rheumatoid arthritis. In addition, Tai Chi has statistically significant benefits on lower extremity range of motion, in particular ankle range of motion, for people with RA. The included studies did not assess the effects on patient-reported pain.

The objective of this systematic review (25) is to evaluate data from controlled clinical trials testing the effectiveness of Tai Chi for treating rheumatoid arthritis (RA). Systematic searches were conducted on Medline, Pubmed, AMED, British Nursing Index, CINAHL, EMBASE, PsycInfo, The Cochrane Library 2007, Issue 1, the UK National Research Register and ClinicalTrials.gov, Korean medical databases, Qigong and Energy Medicine Database and Chinese databases up to January 2007.

Collectively this evidence is not convincing enough to suggest that Tai Chi is an effective treatment for RA. The value of Tai Chi for this indication therefore remains unproven.

Reduction of Anxiety and Depression

In (20), significant improvements in trait anxiety, pain perception, mood, flexibility, and balance were obtained. These may have a profound effect on the incidence of falls, injuries, resulting disability, and overall quality of life.

The study (22) aimed to assess the usefulness of two interventions in a group rehabilitation medicine setting and to determine strategies and exercise guidelines for long-term care of the HIV/AIDS population with human immunodeficiency virus (HIV) and/or acquired immunodeficiency syndrome (AIDS). It concluded that that Tai Chi and exercise improve physiologic parameters, functional outcomes, and quality of life. Group intervention provides a socialization context for management of chronic HIV disease. Further long and short term studies are required.

The effects on blood pressure, lipid profile, and anxiety status on subjects in a 12-week Tai Chi Chuan exercise program were studied (23). It concluded that Tai Chi exercise training could decrease blood pressure and results in favorable lipid profile changes and improve subjects' anxiety status. Therefore, Tai Chi could be used as an alternative modality in treating patients with mild hypertension, with a promising economic effect.

Another paper on the beneficial effect of Tai Chi on depression in older individuals appears in (26).

Immunity

At rest the total number of T-lymphocytes and the number of active T-lymphocytes were increased significantly in the exercise group compared with the controls (8). Immediately after a bout of Tai Chi (88 style), a marked increase of active T-lymphocytes occurred. In conclusion, the results indicate that frequent Tai Chi exercise causes an increase of T-lymphocytes in the blood.

According to a new study (24), Tai Chi may help older adults avoid getting shingles by increasing immunity to varicella-zoster virus (VZV) and boosting the immune response to varicella vaccine in older adults. Tai Chi alone was found to increase participants' immunity to varicella as much as the vaccine typically produces in 30- to 40-year-old adults, and Tai Chi combined with the vaccine produced a significantly higher level of immunity, about a 40 percent increase, over that produced by the vaccine alone. The studies also showed that the Tai Chi group's rate of increase in immunity, over the course of the 25-week study, was double that of the health education (control) group. The Tai Chi and health education groups' VZV immunity had been similar when the study began. In addition, the Tai Chi group reported significant improvements in physical functioning, bodily pain, vitality and mental health. Both groups showed significant declines in the severity of depressive symptoms.

Previous studies have suggested that Tai Chi may improve immune function. This study (27) was intended to examine whether 5 months of moderate Tai Chi and Qigong (TQ) practice could improve the immune response to influenza vaccine in older adults. It concluded that traditional TQ practice improves the antibody response to influenza vaccine in older adults. However, further study is needed to determine whether the enhanced response is sufficient to provide definitive protection from influenza infection.

Balance

Tai Chi can improve balance in the elderly and Parkinson's patients, thus avoiding injuries from falls (29).

References

1. Eisen, M. Qigong and Taiji application in stress management. Part 2: Qigong for stress, Qi Dao, Jan. – Feb., 2008.

2. Achiron, A., Barak, Y., Stern, Y., Noy, S. Electrical sensation during Tai-Chi practice as the first manifestation of multiple sclerosis. Clinical Neurology and Neurosurgery, 99, 280-281, 1997.

3. Sandlund, E. S., & Norlander, T. The effects of Tai Chi Chuan relaxation and exercise on stress responses and well-being: An overview of research. International Journal of Stress Management,7(2), 139–149, April 2000.

4. Wang, C. C., Collet, J. P., & Lau, J. The effect of Tai Chi on health outcomes in patients with chronic conditions. Archive of Internal Medicine, 164, 493–501, 2004.

5. Kuramoto, A. M. Therapeutic benefits of Tai Chi exercise: research review. WMI, 6, 105(7), 42-6, Oct. 2006.

6. Song, R., Lee, E.O., Lam. P. Bae, S.C. Effects of a Sun-style Tai Chi exercise on arthritic symptoms, motivation and the performance of health behaviors in women with osteoarthritis. Taehan Kanho Hakhoe Chi, 37(2),249-56, March 2007.

7. Jin, P.. Changes in heart rate, noradrenaline, cortisol and mood during Tai Chi. Journal of Psychosomatic Research, Vol. 33, No. 2, 197-206, 1989.

8. Sun, X., Xu Y., Xia Y. Determination of E-rosette-forming lymphocytes in aged subjects with Taichiquan exercise. Int. J. Sports med, Vol.10, No 3, 217-219, 1989.

9. Jin, P. Efficacy of Tai Chi, brisk walking, meditation, and reading in reducing mental and emotional stress. Journal of Psychosomatic Research, Vol. 36, No. 4, 361-370, 1992.

10. Lai, J., Lan, C., Wong, M., and Teng, S. Two-year trends in cardiorespiratory function among older Tai Chi Chuan practitioners and sedentary subjects. Journal of the American Geriatric Society, Vol. 43: 1222-1227, 1995.

11. Young, D.R., Appel, L.J., Jee, S. The effects of aerobic exercise and T'ai Chi on blood pressure in the elderly. Circulation v. 97(#8), 54-P54, March 3, 1998.

12. Gong, L, Qian J., Zhang J., Yang Q., Jiang J., and Tao Q. Changes in heart rate and electrocardiogram during Taijiquan exercise; analysis by telemetry in 100 subjects. Chinese Medical Journal 94(9), 589-592, 1981.

13. Channer, K.S., Barrow, D., Barrow, R., Osborne, M., and Ives, G. Changes in haemodynamic parameters following Tai Chi Chuan and aerobic exercise in patients recovering from acute myocardial infarction. Postgraduate Medical Journal, 349-351, 1990.

14. Lee, K.Y. and Jeong, O. Y. The effect of Tai Chi movement in patients with rheumatoid arthritis. Taehan Kanho Hakhoe Chi, 36(2), 278-85, 2006.

15. Lee, H.Y. Comparison of effects among Tai-Chi exercise, aquatic exercise, and a self-help program for patients with knee osteoarthritis. Taehan Kanho Hakhoe Chi, 36(3), 571-80, 2006.

16. Kirsteins, A.E.; Dietz, F.; Hwang, S.M. Evaluating the safety and potential use of a weight-bearing exercise, Tai-Chi Chuan, for rheumatoid arthritis patients. Am. J. Phys. Med. Rehabil., 70(3), 136-41, 1991.

17. Han, A., Robinson, V., Judd, M., Taixiang, W., Wells G.; Tugwell, P. Tai Chi for treating rheumatoid arthritis. Cochtane Database Syst. Rev., (3), CD004859, 2004.

18. Taylor-Piliae, R.E., Haskell, W.L., Waters, C.M.; Froelicher, E.S. J. Adv. Nurs., 54(3), 313-29, 2006.

19. Mustata, S., Cooper, L., Langrick, N., Simon, N., Jassal, S.V,; Oreopoulos, D.G.   The effect of a Tai Chi exercise program on quality of life in patients on peritoneal dialysis: a pilot study. Perit. Dial. Int., 25(3), 291 – 4, 2005.

20. Ross, M.C., Bohannon, A.S., Davis, D.C.; Gurchiek, L. The effects of a short-term exercise program on movement, pain, and mood in the elderly. Results of a pilot study. J. Holist. Nurs., Jun;17(2):139-47, 1999.

21 Audette, J.F., Jin, Y.S. , Newcomer, R., Stein, L. Duncan G., Duncan, G.; frontera, W.R. Tai Chi versus brisk walking in elderly women. Age Aging.   Jul;35(4),388-93, 2006.

22. Galantino, M.L., Shepard, K., Krafft, L., Laperriere, A., Ducette, J., Sorbello, A., Barnish, M., Condoluci, D.; Farrar JT. The effect of group aerobic exercise and t'ai chi on functional outcomes and quality of life for persons living with acquired immunodeficiency syndrome. J. Altern. Complement. Med.   Dec. 11(6),1085-9, 2005.

23. Tsai JC, Wang WH, Chan P, Lin LJ, Wang CH, Tomlinson status in a randomized controlled trial. J. Altern. Complement Med. Oct. 9(5):747-54, 2003.

24. Irwin, M.R., et al. Augmenting immune responses to varicella zoster virus in older adults: A randomized, controlled trial of Tai Chi. Journal of the American Geriatrics Society, Volume 55, 4, 511–517, April 2007.

25. Lee et al. Tai chi for rheumatoid arthritis: systematic review. Rheumatology (Oxford), Nov., 46(11), 1648-51, 2007.

26. Chou, K.L., Lee, P.W., Yu, E.C., Macfarlane, D., Cheng, Y.H., Chan, S.S.; Chi, I. Effect of Tai Chi on depressive symptoms amongst Chinese older patients with depressive disorders: a randomized clinical trial. Int. J. Geriatr. Psychiatry, Nov. 19(11):1105-7, 2004.

27. Yang Y, et al. Effects of a Taiji and Qigong intervention on the antibody response to influenza vaccine in older adults. Am J Chin Med. 35(4), 597-607, 2007.

28. Sato, S., et al.   Effect of Tai Chi training on baroreflex sensitivity and heart rate variability in patients with coronary heart disease. Int. Heart J., 51(4): 238-41, July 2010.

29. Leung, D. P., et al. Tai chi as an intervention to improve balance and reduce falls in older adults: A systematic and meta-analytical review. Altern. Ther. Health Med. 2011 Jan-Feb;17(1):40-8.

Chapter 4

What Is Qigong?

Dr. Mehmet Oz, MD, heart surgeon and the star of the TV show "The Doctor OZ Show" stated, "If you want to be healthy and live to 100, do Qigong." Dr. Oz was not just making wild speculations. Recent research has found a way to predict and increase your life span. Tips of chromosomes are called telomeres. These protective caps, made of repetitive chunks of DNA, keep the rest of the gene-laden chromosomes from disastrously unraveling. Telomeres length has been linked to life span. Longer telomeres have been associated with longer lives and vice versa. A cell's telomeres shorten a bit each time that the cell divides. Telomeres length is decreased by stress and can be increased by reducing stress! Qigong reduces stress. Qigong and its effects are discussed below.

Is strenuous exercise necessary for health?

No. Good physical condition is required for competing athletes and does not insure good health. A trained athlete can have cancer and die from a heart attack. Arnold Schwarzenegger needs to have a heart valve replaced. Strenuous exercise produces toxins and free radicals, which can harm the body. Most people do not have enough time to train properly and so rapid movements can injure muscles and joints. Repetitive strain can lead to chronic injuries and disease. Slow, non-strenuous Qigong can improve your health.

What is Qigong?

The main divisions of modern Qigong (Chi Kung) are: Spiritual, Medical, Martial and Athletic depending on the main goal of the practitioner. However, there is an overlap between these branches.

Medical Qigong is a branch of Traditional Chinese Medicine (TCM). Qi can be translated as life energy. TCM postulates that health is the result of smooth Qi circulation, without accumulation or deficiency in any part of the body, while disease is the result of poor Qi circulation. Once the flow of Qi is balanced, the body tends to heal itself. A diagnosis must be made and the proper type of Qigong prescribed.

In Chinese "Gong" means work or hard task. Qigong is the task of learning to control the flow of Qi through your body by using breath, movement and meditation. If you are taught genuine Qigong, passed down from master to disciple, the only requirement for success is dedication and practice.

Why study Qigong?

Some reasons for studying Qigong are: stress relief, relaxation, mental improvement, preventing and self-healing of diseases, spiritual enlightenment; harmony with nature and developing esoteric powers. It is the key to inner power, stamina and resistance to injury in Chinese Martial Arts. Chinese athletes use it to reach peak performance levels. Qigong can increase longevity and improve the quality of life as one ages.

Another reason is to become a Qigong therapist. Diseases can be treated in two ways. The therapist can prescribe Qigong exercise for a particular disease or he can inject his Qi to treat the disease. In Chinese Qigong hospitals both methods are used simultaneously. A therapist should learn several different Qigong methods in order to treat different diseases and to accommodate patients.

Can athletes, couch potatoes or handicapped people benefit from Qigong?

Yes. They are easy to learn requiring very little coordination. They are suitable for the young, old, strong, weak, and infirm, because they can be practiced standing, seated or lying. No equipment, special clothing or partners are required. There is no restriction on the place or time of their performance.

There are dynamic Qigong exercises that will satisfy the most robust people. Athletes can use Qigong not only to improve their peak performance, but also to speed recovery from strenuous training and ameliorate deleterious effects such as lactic acid build up, free radicals etc.

Individual programs can be constructed to aid recovery from illness or injury. It is has been shown that Qigong plus other forms of therapy (western or TCM) works better than Qigong or therapy alone.

Is Qigong scientific?

Conferences on the scientific study of Qigong have been held in the U.S. and China. Qigong has been shown to improve respiration, induce the relaxation response, cause favorable changes in blood chemistry, and produce changes in EEG indicating improved mental states.

Clinical trials have shown the efficacy of Qigong in reducing stress, delaying aging effects, prolonging life, preventing illness and helping to cure about 200 diseases, including paralysis and cancer. The interested reader can find references in the book by Liu, T., Chen, K. et al., Eds. Chinese Medical Qigong. Singing Dragon, London, 2010.

Does Qigong Have Anti-Aging Effects?

Yes. For example, one survey of aged practitioners revealed that they were in good health and appeared younger than a second group of non-practitioners. Their average blood pressure was normal and 93% had normal hearing and good memories. The non-practicing elders had a higher average blood pressure, 25% had hypertension, 50% had vision problems, 76% had hearing problems and 35% had lost their ability to work. After doing Qigong for 5 months, 52% of them recovered some of their working ability and made other physiological improvements.

When being treated by external Qi does the patient have to move or feel it to be cured?

No. Some people feel the effects of the Qi or move. Others do not feel anything and do not move. Both classes of people can benefit. Studies have shown that there is no correlation between the movements of the therapist and the patient.

Can a "Master" inject Qi and open all of your channels to give you powers or permanently improve your health?

Be suspicious of such a claim especially if the "Master" asks for a large sum of money. If you get a bowl of rice today you will feel good, but tomorrow you will feel hungry. The "gong" in Qigong stands for hard work. There is no royal road to learning. A standard recommendation is that you must practice 100 days in a row to obtain some benefit. If you miss one day you must start over, even if that day was the 99th.

How many forms of Qigong are there?

There are about 3000 different forms of Qigong. The different styles can be divided into three classes: medical, martial, and spiritual. These divisions overlap. However, to really become proficient in one branch you must specialize in that type of Qigong. For example, a spiritual practitioner can have developed tremendous amounts of Qi but can still be mediocre in applications to the martial arts.

Is Tai Chi a form of Qigong?

Yes. In the beginning Tai Chi seems to be a physical exercise. Later, with proper instruction, you will realize it is a form of Qigong. Each posture affects certain organs and can be used to heal diseases. After a long time you can feel the effects of your Qi during movements. There are also martial applications of Qi, since Tai Chi is a martial as well as a healing art. Tai Chi is a very difficult form of Qigong to learn.

Can Qigong endanger your life?

Some hospitals have so-called Qigong classes for patients with serious illnesses, such as cancer. Patients are encouraged to drop in to these classes, when they come for treatment. Such programs might make you feel good, but are not effective for treating serious diseases. Patients are not told that this is not enough time to spend or even the right type of Qigong for their problem, which requires a proper diagnosis by a Medical Qigong doctor. In China, patients treated with Qigong practice 3 to 6 hours daily.

Chapter 5

Senobi Breathing for Reducing Obesity, Symptoms of Asthma and Depression

The Senobi Breathing Method can be done sitting or standing. The hands are extended above the head with the palms upward. (Fingers are intertwined or not). Lean back and arch the neck backwards. Inhale for 5 seconds and then exhale for 5 seconds. Repeat this breathing cycle 6 times. This is done before every meal. Use abdominal breathing as described in the next two paragraphs.

Abdominal breathing can be practiced lying down or sitting in a chair. The practice methods are similar. The method of practice while sitting in a chair will be described. Inhale and exhale gently, smoothly and continuously through your nose.

Sit comfortably, with your knees bent and your shoulders, head and neck relaxed. Place one hand on your upper chest and the other just below your rib cage. This will allow you to feel your diaphragm move as you breathe. On inhalation, the hand on your chest must move as little as possible, while the hand on your abdomen must move outwards. On exhalation, the hand on your abdomen moves inward. This movement can be helped by slightly and gently pulling your abdominal muscle inward. Once again, the hand on your chest moves as little as possible. At first, you'll probably get tired while doing this exercise because an increased effort will be needed to use the diaphragm correctly. Keep at it, because with continued practice, abdominal breathing will become easy and automatic.

The study (1) found significant losses in body fat after 1 month of regular practice. Using various measures researchers found substantial up-regulation of sympathetic nerve activity and increased urinary hormone secretion after 1 min of the Senobi breathing method. They did not find these results in the non-obese control group.

Psychological factors can also be involved in obesity such as: stress, depression, poor food choices, not realizing the discrepancy between calorie intake and calories burned by activity, etc. Practicing additional abdominal breathing for relaxation and stress relief and reflecting on the food you eat may lead to additional weight loss.

The researchers in (2) used heart rate variability measurements to determine levels of parasympathetic (rest and digest) nerve dominance. Higher levels of parasympathetic control are thought to lead to asthma symptoms as the sympathetic nervous system (fight or flight) is in control of opening the airway passages.

Asthmatic patients were asked to engage in the Senobi breathing exercise regularly for 1 month. At the conclusion of this month the majority of patients showed a decrease in use of their inhalers and showed an increase in expiratory volume. Senobi breathing is thought to activate the sympathetic nervous system thus opening airway passages.

Obese individuals have an increased risk of developing depression. The study (3) showed that after one month "Senobi" breathing could relieve depression, especially in obese women.

Hopefully, these applications of Senobi breathing will sway readers to consider that strenuous exercise is not necessary for health improvement and arouse their curiosity to explore Qigong for longevity and combating many diseases.

References

1. Sato, K. et al. The "Senobi" breathing exercise is recommended as first line treatment for obesity. Biomed. Res., (4):259-62, 2010.
2. Sato, K., et al. "Senobi" stretch ameliorates asthma symptoms by restoring autonomic nervous system balance. J. Investig. Med. 58(8):968-70, 2010.
3. Sato, K., et al. The "Senobi" breathing exercise ameliorates depression in obese women through up-regulation of sympathetic nerve activity and hormone secretion. Biomed. Res. 32(2):175-80, 2011.

Chapter 6

Using Qigong Breathing Exercises to Relieve Hypertension, an Enlarged Prostate or Arrhythmias

High blood pressure is frequently difficult to treat in a short time by acupuncture or herbs. Patients become discouraged and turn to western medicine. Some forms of Qigong can help lower blood pressure. However, most of these forms must be taught to the patient and are not simple to learn.

Most of these Qigong methods have a common factor. The rate of respiration is slowed down. This may be the chief parameter which accounts for their lowering of blood pressure.

Recent research shows that 3 or 4 15-minute sessions of slow breathing (less than or equal to 10 breaths per minute) can lower both systolic and diastolic blood pressure, usually within 8 weeks (1) – (19). Breathing exercises should be practiced about a half an hour daily. In one clinical trial, some diabetics were not able to sufficiently lower their respiration rate. However, with a longer training period a lower rate of respiration might be achieved.

The breathing exercise should be performed using so-called abdominal, normal, Buddhist or diaphragmatic breathing, like opera singers. The Daoists thought that normal breathing was one of the secrets of longevity. If you look at a baby in its crib you will only notice its stomach move up and down as it breathes. By contrast, when most seniors breathe their upper chest heaves up and down and there is no visible movement of their abdomen, a consequence of shallow breathing. A Chinese doctor looks at the abdomen of a critically ill patient. If it moves up and down as the patient breathes, the patient has a better chance of surviving than a patient with no visible abdominal movement on breathing. Thus, you may have to instruct patients so that normal or diaphragmatic breathing is done automatically.

Normal or diaphragmatic breathing can be practiced lying down or sitting in a chair. The practice methods are similar. The method of practice while sitting in a chair will be described. Inhale and exhale gently, smoothly and continuously through your nose. Sit comfortably, with your knees bent and your shoulders, head and neck relaxed. Place one hand on your upper chest and the other just below your rib cage. This will allow you to feel your diaphragm move as you breathe. On inhalation, the hand on your chest must move as little as possible, while the hand on your abdomen must move outwards. On exhalation, the hand on your abdomen moves inward. Once again, the hand on your chest moves as little as possible. At first, you'll probably get tired while doing this exercise because an increased effort will be needed to use the diaphragm correctly. Keep at it, because with continued practice, diaphragmatic breathing will become easy and automatic. Practice this exercise 5-10 minutes a few times a day.

Slow breathing has the physiological effect of relaxing the muscles surrounding the small blood vessels, which allows the blood to flow more easily. Alpha blockers block receptors in arteries and smooth muscle. This action relaxes the blood vessels and leads to an increase in blood flow and a lower pressure for the control of hypertension. The action in the urinary tract enhances urinary flow for an enlarged prostate. Slow breathing seems to have the same effect as alpha blockers. Thus, it may also reduce the symptoms of an enlarged prostate. This conjecture has not been subjected to clinical trials, but has worked on one subject.

There is another simple breathing technique purported to help eliminate and prevent heart attacks due to abnormal electrical events to the heart, and to generally enhance performance of the central nervous system (CNS) and to help eliminate the effects of traumatic shock and stress to the CNS. Most patients would prefer to try this approach rather than the risks of ablation or a cardiac pacemaker.

The method requires 1 breath per minute (BPM) respiratory exercise with slow inspiration for 20 seconds, breath retention for 20 seconds, and slow expiration for 20 seconds, for 31 consecutive minutes. Do not attempt to use the required time intervals to start. Use a time interval - say, 5 seconds, or even less, so that no straining is involved. Try to practice every day for 30 minutes.

This technique produced favorable shifts in all hemodynamic variables measured for 4 subjects during the 1 BPM exercise and in the post-exercise resting period (20). The authors conclude that the long-term effects of this technique appear to reset a cardio-respiratory brain-stem pacemaker. This effect may be the basis for the purported health claim of this yogic breathing exercise. Large scale clinical trials seem warranted.

References

1. Device-Guided Breathing to Lower Blood Pressure: Case Report and Clinical Overview. W Elliott, J Izzo. Medscape General Medicine, 2006; 8(3).

2. Graded Blood Pressure Reduction in Hypertensive Outpatients Associated with Use of a Device to Assist with Slow Breathing. W Elliott, J Izzo, Jr., WB White, D Rosing, CS Snyder, A Alter, B Gavish, HR Black, J. Clin. Hypertens., 2004 6(10): 553-559.

3. Nonpharmacologic Treatment of Hypertension by Respiratory Exercise in the Home Setting. E Meles, C Giannattasio, M Failla, G Gentile, A Capra, G Mancia, American Journal of Hypertension 2004, 17:370–374.

4. Respiration and Blood Pressure. G Parati, JL Izzo Jr, B Gavish, in Hypertension Primer, Third Edition. JL Izzo and HR Black, Eds. Baltimore, Lippincott, Williams, and Wilkins, 2003; Ch. A40, p117-120.

5. Non-Pharmacological Treatment of Resistant Hypertensives by Device-Guided Slow Breathing Exercises. R Viskoper , I Shapira, R Priluck, R Mindlin, L Chornia, A Laszt, D Dicker, B Gavish, A Alter, American Journal of Hypertension 2003; Vol. 16:484-487.

6. Device-Guided Breathing Exercises Reduce Blood Pressure - Ambulatory and Home Measurements. T Rosenthal, A Alter, E Peleg, B Gavish, American Journal of Hypertension 2001; 14:74-76.

7. Breathing-control lowers blood pressure.E Grossman, A Grossman , MH Schein, R Zimlichman, B Gavish. Journal of Human Hypertension 2001; 15:263-269.

8. Treating hypertension with a device that slows and regularizes breathing: A randomised, double-blind controlled study. M Schein, B Gavish, M Herz , D Rosner-Kahana, P Naveh, B Knishkowy, E Zlotnikov, N Ben-Zvi, RN Melmed , Journal of Human Hypertension 2001; 15:271-278.

9. The Changes of Noninvasive Hemodynamic Parameters after Device-Guided Slow Breathing Exercise in Hypertensive Patients. J Y Kim, M S Han, H H Yoo, H M Choe, B S Yoo, S H Lee, J Yoon, and K H Choe. Journal of Clinical Hypertension,2006, Vol 8, Issue 5, Suppl A.

10. Does Baseline Systolic Blood Pressure Affect Antihypertensive Efficacy with Device-Guided Breathing Exercise? Kim JY, Han MS, Yoo HH, Choe HM, Yoo BS, Lee SH, Yoon J, and Choe KH. Journal of Clinical Hypertension,2006, Volume 8, Issue 5, Suppl. A.

11. Non-pharmacological treatment of hypertension in diabetics by device-guided paced breathing: A randomized controlled study. M H Schein, A Alter and B Gavish. Journal of Clinical Hypertension, 2006, Vol. 8, Issue 5, Supl. A,. P- 79.

12. Blood pressure change following 8-week, 15-minute daily treatment with paced breathing guided by a device: A Korean multi-center study. J H Bae, J H Kim, K H Choe, S P Hong, K S Kim, C H Kim and W H Kim. Journal of Clinical Hypertension,2006, Vol. 8, Issue 5, Suppl. A,. P-86

13. Treating hypertension in diabetics with device-guided breathing: A randomized controlled study. MH Schein, A Alter and B Gavish. EGPRN 2005.

14. Treating high blood pressure by device-guided paced breathing in the home setting: Evidence-based approach. M Schein, E Grossman, T Rosenthal, C Giannattasio, W Elliott, R Viskoper, A Alter, B Gavish British Hypertension Society Annual Meeting, Cambridge, UK. Sept 2005

15. Reduction of home blood pressures and white coat effect after 8 weeks of device-guided paced breathing. W Elliott, B Gavish, A Alter, J L. Izzo, and H R. Black, American Journal of Hypertension, 2005, 18(5): 211A

16. Blood pressure reduction with device-guided breathing: Pooled data from 7 controlled studies. Elliott, HR Black, A Alter, B Gavish. Journal of Hypertension, 2004; 22(2): S116

17. Acute effects of device guided-breathing on cardiovascular parameters and baroreflex sensitivity in normal subjects. G Parati, F Glavina, G Ongaro, A Maronati, B Gavish, P Castiglioni, M Di Rienzo, G Mancia. American Journal of Hypertension, 2002; 15(4,2)182A.

18. The pressure dependence of arterial compliance: A model interpretation. B Gavish, American Journal of Hypertension, 2001; 14:121A. 2004; 17(5):54A

19. Are breathing exercises an active component in reducing high blood pressure? A retrospective view. B Gavish. Journal of Hypertension 2001, Supplement 2, S79-S80.

Repeated blood pressure measurements may probe directly an arterial property. Gavish B., American Journal of Hypertension 2000; 13:190A.

20. Hemodynamic Observations on a Yogic Breathing Technique Claimed to Help Eliminate and Prevent Heart Attacks: A Pilot Study. David S. Shannahoff, Khalsa, B., Bo Sramek, Matthew B. Kennel, Stuart W. Jamieson, J. of Alternative and Complementary Medicine, Volume 10, Number 5, 2004, pp.757 -766.

Chapter 7

Should You Study Yoga, Tai Chi or Qigong?

Yoga and Tai Chi have become popular worldwide. They appear in commercials and are taught in many fitness and community centers. Seniors and the sedentary are persuaded that Yoga and Tai Chi are ideal for their health. In addition, Tai Chi is described as being very easy to learn and practice. Not as many people are familiar with Qigong, a coordinated mind, body, breathing discipline which originated in China thousands of years ago.

These arts have become westernized, commercialized and altered from their original purposes and forms. You should study, learn and research about the history, theory, safety and true purposes of these arts before choosing one of these disciplines to study. Many medical professionals have erroneous ideas about Yoga, Tai Chi and Qigong,

There are hardly any Yoga teachers that teach Yoga for its originally intended purpose. Yoga had no connection with health, but was just a spiritual discipline; you could not pay for true Yoga lessons – see Chapter 2.

Be careful in practicing Yoga poses, especially seniors and the sedentary; don't believe the so-called experts. See its dangers described in the reference in Chapter 2

Unfortunately, Tai Chi is following the same path as Yoga. Originally Tai Chi was a martial art and had over 100 postures. This main, solo long form required about 5 to six years of dedicated practice to learn correctly. In addition, there were 2- men formulas for self-defense – see Chapter 3.

Nowadays, there are very few teachers that know the 2-men, self-defense forms or even a classical Tai Chi form. Many well- meaning teachers have been taught by teachers that teach Tai Chi solely for profit and so cannot be strict and have to amuse their students. Even those that teach Tai Chi for health don't rigorously follow the principles (Appendix) and claim that the form they teach (1- 37 postures or more, but usually less than the long form) has the same benefits as the long form. Logic tells you that 37 postures will not give the same exercise and energy flow as over a hundred.

Even teaching the Chen Man Ching short form for health correctly is difficult. The student must have the dedication of a ballet dancer and realize constant daily practice is required. After teaching 100's of students, less than 1% can even learn this short form. The reasons are that they don't practice at home, can't memorize the principles (Appendix) and moves and don't have a burning desire to learn. You must have perseverance and not give up even though you make mistakes. It is like memorizing an English poem. At first, you only remember a few lines and even those not correctly. However, after many repetitions, you finally learn it.

Prospective Tai Chi students should be informed of the true scope of this art. Most don't have any idea of the complexities of Tai Chi and are just interested in improving their health. Advanced students must study Traditional Chinese medical theory besides the forms. This theory I required to understand the health aspects produced by each move and to strike vital points for self-defense.

Seniors and the sedentary, especially if only interested in improving or maintaining their health, should learn and practice Qigong (See Chapter 4.) for health rather than Yoga or Tai Chi.   My experience is that nearly 100% of students can learn such Qigong forms

Qigong is non-strenuous and easier to learn and practice than Yoga or Tai Chi. It can be done lying, sitting or standing. Qigong requires no special equipment, uniforms or a great deal of room and so can be done anywhere. It can help about 200 diseases, ranging from the common cold to cancer. Qigong has the added advantage that it can teach you how to cultivate your Qi and how to utilize it for not only maintaining health, but to help heal oneself. In addition, it can, with advanced study, be utilized to heal others.

Appendix

Some Basic Principles for Doing Yang Tai Chi

1. Relax (Sung) but don't collapse (shoulders and elbows down; sink chest).

2. Sink (Chen).

3. Back straight:

(a)   Nose and navel lined up. However, your eyes must look in the direction of your final position, where the imaginary opponent would be. Tai Chi also exercises the eyes.

(b)   Eliminate the curve in the lower back by tucking the tail bone under. Imagine a weight attached to the tail bone and relax. Use relaxation and gravity; not muscle power.

(c)   Head held up as if suspended from the top by a string.

4. Turn but don't twist. The turning is initiated from your center. The whole body turns at once from toe to head about a center line passing straight down from your head to your perineum.

5. Originally, Yang was interpreted as the sunny side of a mountain and Yin the dark side. Yin and Yang became two complementary principles of Chinese philosophy. Yin is dark, negative, passive, un-weighted, relaxed, feminine, etc. Yang is bright, positive, masculine, active, weighted, masculine, etc. Nothing is completely Yin or Yang. These are extremes, which can change. Their interaction is thought to maintain the harmony of the universe and to influence everything within it. These principles must be applied in Tai Chi. For example: avoiding double weighting, by learning the amount of weight on each foot, memorizing the relative amounts of tension in various parts of your body, etc.

6. Tai Chi (ladies') hands.

7. Don't move the hands or feet by themselves. Use turning of the waist and hips from your center for side motions, gravity for downward motions and sinking for upward motions.

8. Don't grip the floor with your toes. Relax your foot and ankle and let your weight go down into the heart of your foot.

9. Use abdominal breathing. Don't try to breath- in a fixed manner but relax and breathe naturally. Eventually you till breath correctly because of the movement produced by the exercise.

10. Move slowly and imagine the air to be a thick liquid. Try to feel the air.

11. The Tai Chi form is performed slowly and continuously at a constant rate of speed as if pulling silk from a cocoon.

12. Touch the heel when stepping forward and the ball of the foot when stepping backward.

13. Elbows point to the ground and are slightly below the hand in ward off.

14. When you are moving keep your head at the same level; don't bob.

15. Transfer your weight slowly to the leg with no weight. Think of an hour glass being turned over. The sand gradually falls from the top to the bottom. All of the sand does not appear suddenly in the bottom container.

www.ingramcontent.com/pod-product-compliance
Lightning Source LLC
Chambersburg PA
CBHW080356290526
45791CB00009BA/2901